I0421291

Natural Remedies that Heal!

Natural Remedies

Ancient Primordial Cures, Treatments And Home Remedies To Protect Yourself And Provide Instant Relief From Everyday Common Ailments!

Mia Conrad

Copyright © 2014 Mia Conrad

STOP!!! Before you read any further....Would you like to know the secrets of Anti-Aging?

If your answer is yes, then you are not alone. Thousands of people are looking for the secret to reducing wrinkles, looking younger, and maintaining a youthful appearance.

If you have been searching for these answers without much luck, you are in the right place!

Not only will you gain incredible insight in this book, but because I want to make sure to give you as much value as possible, right now for a limited time you can get full **100% FREE access to a VIP bonus EBook** entitled **Anti-Aging Made Easy!**

Just Go Here For Free Instant Access:

www.LuxyLifeNaturals.com

Legal Notice

Disclaimer Notice

Table Of Contents

Introduction

I want to thank you and congratulate you for purchasing the book "Natural Remedies – Ancient Primordial Cures, Treatments, And Home Remedies To Protect Yourself And Provide Instant Relief From Everyday Common Ailments!"

This "Natural Remedies" book contains proven steps and strategies on how to treat a variety of health conditions using natural remedies. In this book, you will learn about the different herbs and plants that can help you improve your condition. You will also learn about the history of herbal remedies and why they are better than traditional medicines.

Today, more and more people are realizing the benefits of alternative medicine. This is great because natural treatments are generally less invasive and more cost-effective than prescription and over-the-counter drugs. If you want to feel better without experiencing negative side effects, you should look into these natural remedies.

Thanks again for purchasing this book, I hope you enjoy it!

Chapter 1: History Of Natural Remedies

Herbal medicine is one of the oldest forms of medicine. In fact, it has been used by people since the beginning of time. Today, there are still systems of herbal medicine that remain in use, such as Traditional Chinese Herbal Medicine and Ayurveda that originated from India. Both of these systems make use of herbal combinations. In the West, however, herbal medicine focuses more on simple or individual herbs.

Herbal medicine is still used by about eighty percent of people all over the world. Elements of trees, shrubs, and plants are prepared as teas, poultices, and extracts. Herbs are actually the foundation of modern pharmacology. They have been used to produce modern forms of medicine. Morphine, for instance, is derived from poppy while aspirin is derived from the herb white willow back.

Similarly, a lot of medicines used to fight cancer are derived from herbs such as parsley, Madagascar periwinkle, and rosemary; but when did herbal medicines become prominent? Well, according to old records from the 1500 BC, the ancient Egyptians used juniper, myrrh, and garlic for medicinal purposes. In 1000 AD, herbs were used by the people of England to protect themselves against infections.

During the Middle Ages, the citizens of Britain used herbs that they believed were 'signed' by God. Milk thistle, for example, was believed to be beneficial for nursing mothers due to the milk-like stains on its leaves. Dandelions were also believed to be ideal for jaundice due to the yellow color of their flowers. All throughout Europe, herbal medicine was also believed to be used by witches.

Since the thirteenth century, numerous women have been accused of using herbs for witchcraft. Men from medical schools and barber-surgeon guilds have also displaced traditional female herbalists. In the nineteenth century, chemistry has enabled people to use herbs better. Active ingredients were extracted from herbs, and the French word 'drogue' meaning 'herb' became the term for chemical drugs.

In America, herbal medicine first became popular when Samuel Thompson disapproved of the side effects of traditional medicine. He started the 'root and herb' medicinal approach, which was eventually brought by Albert Coffin to Britain. The National Association of Medicinal Herbalists was founded in 1864 and was renamed the National Institute of Medicinal Herbalists in 1945.

There have also been many women who became notable for their help in establishing herbal medicine. Abbess Hildegard, a German teacher, physician, and musician; Trotula, chairwoman of Salerno Medical School; Hilda Leyel, founder of the Herb Society; and Maud Grieve, a promoter of herbal medicine during World War I, were some of them.

In Southeast Asian and Indian cultures, herbal medicine is also prominent. In fact, they have been using herbs for over six thousand years. Early tribal societies chewed on herbs and grasses to relieve stomachaches. Ayurvedic medicine was also used for healing. It is actually a tradition that began in the Hindu religion and focuses on following the strategies and principles for good health and long life.

The Chinese used herbs to treat ailments and balance energies. In Egyptian and Greek cultures, plants and herbs were also used for medicinal purposes. Today, herbs are still widely used for healing. Modern medical herbalists train for several years and do scientific research. They study medicinal sciences, pharmacy, botany and nutrition among others.

Chapter 2: Why Natural Alternatives vs. Prescription Drugs

If you are not feeling well, you may wonder whether to buy prescription drugs or resort to alternative treatments such as herbal remedies. In the past, people relied on herbs to treat their ailments. Due to the advancements in technology, however, drugs have been produced in laboratories. Physicians prescribe these modern drugs to patients to treat a variety of diseases including cancer and heart disease.

With this being said, should you go for prescription drugs or herbal medicine? Well, you should know that about half of the prescription and over-the-counter drugs available today are derived from herbs and plants. Even though modern drugs are made with chemicals, scientists still incorporate natural compounds. Then again, herbal remedies are not regulated by the Food and Drug Administration (FDA).

Natural treatments are usually not advertised and labeled as legal cures or treatments. Herbal remedies do not offer much statutory protection, which is why they are usually not recommended by doctors. Prescription drugs, on the other hand, are mostly effective because the pharmaceutical companies that manufacture them have already isolated the active ingredients in the plant or herb.

Thus, you can fully benefit from these active ingredients and steer clear from any toxic substances that the plant or herb may contain. Then again, most herbalists disagree with this. They believe that all parts of plants and herbs should be utilized. They believe that isolating active ingredients from plants and herbs also eliminates the vitamins and minerals that they contain.

If you purchase over-the-counter drugs, you can get better but you may also experience unpleasant side effects. According to the AMA Journal, prescription drug side effects are actually the fourth leading cause of death in the United States. More than one hundred thousand individuals die each year due to prescription drugs. About two million people also experience serious side effects from these medications.

If you take all factors into consideration, you will realize that prescription drugs and improper medical treatment are actually the second leading cause of death in the United States. Your condition can improve when you take prescription drugs, but you can also suffer from their side effects. So if you want to play safe, you should go for herbal treatments instead.

You cannot trust the pharmaceutical industry and the FDA one hundred percent anyway. In recent years, there has been several prescription drug recalls. According to a study in 2006, the credibility of health care providers, the pharmaceutical industry, the FDA, and the academic research enterprise has been diminished.

What's more, prescription drugs tend to be very expensive. This is why more and more people are turning to alternative medicines. In fact, in 2001, it has been reported that one in every four senior citizens leave prescriptions unfilled or skip doses. Herbal remedies are much cheaper, which is why they are preferred by more consumers.

Herbal remedies can be just as effective as prescription drugs if used properly. These remedies are also safer and have little or no side effects. However, before you start herbal treatment, see to it that you consult a legitimate herbalist. You should also seek clearance from your doctor to make sure that your new treatment method will not cause any allergic reactions or complications.

Chapter 3: Natural Remedies For Seasonal Ailments

The changes in weather can bring about a variety of ailments. Well, this is not really surprising considering that your body has to adapt to such changes. In the summer, for instance, the weather is hot so your body tries to keep cool. When winter comes, your body has to work hard to keep warm. In the spring, your body has to protect itself against allergens, such as pollen, which is typically present in the atmosphere during this time of the year.

Summer Ailments

Summer is the best time to head to the beach, but it is also the time when sunburns are most common. If you are not able to avoid sunburns, you can use Aloe Vera gel to relieve pain, prevent scars and blisters, and quicken healing. Just break off an Aloe Vera leaf and open it to squeeze out the gel. Then, apply the gel directly to the affected area two times a day. You can also use lavender oil to prevent scarring and speed up healing.

Perspiration and heat can increase your chances of having athlete's foot. If you go out barefoot, there is a higher chance that you will have itchy, cracked, dry, and sore skin. To treat athlete's foot naturally, you can use tea tree oil. This essential oil has antifungal properties. Just combine one-fourth teaspoon of almond oil or olive oil with several drops of tea tree oil and use the mixture to rub on your feet two times a day. Within several days, the itching will stop; but you still need to continue applying it on your feet once a day until the fungus is totally gone.

Bugs and ticks are usually present during the summer. If you are bitten by a bug, you can apply Echinacea tincture directly to your bug bite to alleviate swelling and itching. You can also place several drops of the tincture under your tongue to let you prevent infections. Make it a habit to shower every time after you went outdoors. Inspect your skin for ticks and remove them if you see any.

Winter Ailments

During the winter, your body adjusts to changes in temperature, climate and diet. Because of this, bacteria and viruses start to attack it. Your body becomes susceptible to infections and ailments such as flue, sore throat, cough and cold. Other ailments common during this time of the year include itchy and dry skin, chest congestion, runny noses and seasonal allergies. Those who have asthma and arthritis experience aggravated symptoms.

If you want to find relief from cough, congestion, bronchitis and cold, you can use tea tree oil due to its natural expectorant properties. Just rub it on your chest or put a tiny amount on your pillow so you can inhale it when you sleep. You can also use thyme to treat bronchitis, cough and upper respiratory infections. You can make thyme tea by mixing two teaspoons of crushed thyme leaves in a cup of boiling water. Cover the cup and steep for about ten minutes before straining.

For dry cough, you can drink turmeric tea. Just mix carom seeds with turmeric powder in a cup of boiling water. You can even add honey to strengthen its healing effects. Honey can act as a mild antibiotic. For wet cough with mucus, you can drink black pepper tea. Just combine honey and ground black pepper in a cup of boiling water, cover it for about fifteen minutes, and then strain. If you do not have black pepper, you can substitute it with cayenne. To soothe chapped and cracked skin, you can use natural oils such as avocado, jojoba and coconut.

Spring Ailments

In the spring, you can suffer from seasonal allergies due to the changes in weather and presence of pollen in the air. Hay fever, also called allergic rhinitis, is actually very common during this time. Although not particularly debilitating or life threatening, this ailment can interfere with your daily activities. So when you notice symptoms, including coughing, sneezing, watery eyes, headaches, nasal congestion, and itchiness in the eyes, nose, and throat, you should start treatment.

You can use a saline solution to alleviate congestion and get rid of allergens. Just combine one-fourth teaspoon of salt and two cups of water in a squeeze bottle or neti pot. You can also drink ginger with lime and honey to treat hay fever. Likewise, you can use nettle extracts to improve your condition. Inhaling steam can also be helpful in soothing your nasal passages. Just add several drops of peppermint, lavender or eucalyptus oil to hot water and inhale their vapors.

To help improve your immune system, you can make a Bayberry decoction. It is also ideal to drink green tea since it is high in antioxidants. You can also drink chamomile or peppermint tea to treat ailments associated with your respiratory system. Other home remedies you can use to treat seasonal allergies include apple cider vinegar, reishi mushrooms, turmeric, licorice root and cinnamon. Furthermore, the Herbal Academy of New England suggests goldenrod and elderflower for seasonal allergies.

Chapter 4: Natural Remedies For Skin Ailments

Your skin is the largest organ of your body, which is why it is only proper that you take good care of it. Perhaps the best way to take care of your skin is to have a healthy diet. Keep in mind that what you eat can reflect on the way you look. If you eat nutritious foods, then your entire body will be healthy.

Also, you should take care of your liver because it is the organ responsible for detoxification. If you experience high levels of stress, then your liver can be overburdened because it has to keep up with the needs of your body. If your liver is not able to function optimally, you can develop skin conditions such as acne, rashes and eczema.

So to keep your liver from functioning properly, you should cleanse it. You can use castor oil and alterative tea. Milk thistle is also recommended. It is actually used in treating liver poisoning and liver cirrhosis. It is also effective in protecting the liver against toxins. Dietitians recommend taking milk thistle capsules to support liver cell regeneration.

Eczema or dermatitis is one of the most common skin disorders. It typically causes red, dry, itchy and painful skin. At times, it may even cause bleeding and crusting over. To treat eczema, herbal teas from nettle, albizia, calendula, licorice, and chamomile can be taken. Aloe Vera gel can also be taken internally to reduce inflammation.

Essential oils can also be beneficial for inflamed skin. Lavender, geranium, argan, and chamomile oil can help treat eczema and other skin conditions. However, if you have sensitive skin, you may want to test essential oils by combining them with olive, avocado or any other carrier oil and placing the mixture on your inner wrist.

If you have irritated skin, you can soothe it by taking a chamomile tea bath. If you have dandruff and seborrheic dermatitis, you can use a shampoo with tea tree oil to soothe your scaly and dry scalp as well as prevent hair loss. Tea tree oil is also effective in getting rid of blackheads and whiteheads and disinfecting pores.

A study published in The British Journal of Dermatology even showed that tea tree oil can reduce the severity and amount of acne lesions. So if you have acne, you can clear your skin by applying a five percent tea tree solution to the affected area. Be careful not to use undiluted tea tree oil as it can cause redness, itching, blistering and irritation.

Tea tree oil mixes well with Aloe Vera gel, raw honey and jojoba oil. Tea tree oil mixtures are effective in treating pimples and other blemishes. Moreover, tea tree oil is useful in treating psoriasis, skin tags and warts. The antimicrobial properties of this essential oil can naturally heal your skin.

Chapter 5: Natural Remedies For Gastrointestinal Ailments

Your gastrointestinal tract includes your intestines and stomach. The upper tract consists of your duodenum, esophagus and stomach while the lower tract consists of your large intestine and small intestine. Your gastrointestinal tract releases hormones, such as gastrin, ghrelin, secretin and cholecystokinin, to aid your body in the digestion process.

Normally, it takes about thirty to forty hours for your digested food to pass through your colon or large intestine. Once the food passes through, the digestion cycle is completed. It is crucial for you to take good care of your gastrointestinal tract. Otherwise, you may have serious conditions like appendicitis, abdominal tumors and colorectal cancer. This may require you to undergo surgical procedures.

Then again, not all gastrointestinal tract problems need surgery and other immediate medical procedures. If you experience problems such as irritable bowel syndrome, constipation, indigestion, heartburn, diarrhea, bloating, gastroenteritis, nausea, gastroesophageal reflux disease and gastric ulcers, you can resort to natural treatments including herbal remedies.

Cranberry juice, for instance, is an ideal treatment for urinary tract infections and gastric ulcers. You can also drink Aloe Vera juice if you have irritable bowel syndrome characterized by bloating, constipation, gas, diarrhea and/or abdominal pain. Different kinds of tea are also effective in relieving indigestion and stomach cramps. You can drink green, mint, ginger or fennel tea to reduce flatulence or stomach gas.

Chamomile is useful in treating numerous digestive and stomach ailments, including irritable bowel syndrome, constipation, indigestion, and even menstrual cramps. You can either take chamomile as tea or a supplement. Oilssuch as peppermint and geranium are helpful too.

Peppermint oil is useful in releasing intestinal and stomach gas, as well as in treating stomachaches, bowel spasms and irritable bowel syndrome. Geranium oil, on the other hand, can help get rid of intestinal worms. It is also effective in treating duodenal and stomach ulcers, and throat and nose diseases.

If you have never used barks before, now is the time to use white oak and slippery elm. White oak bark has natural antibacterial properties, which makes it helpful in eliminating parasites from the gastrointestinal tract and preventing infections. Slippery elm bark has soothing properties and is useful in treating gastritis, duodenal ulcers, colitis, heartburn, irritable bowel syndrome and hemorrhoids.

Roots are good for your gastrointestinal tract as well. Dandelion root, for instance, is not only good for digestion but can also reduce habitual constipation and relieve stomachaches. Chicory root can help detoxify your body, regulate your metabolism and purify your blood. It can also treat colitis, gastritis and hemorrhoids. It can even help remove intestinal worms and prevent intestinal cancer.

Licorice root can reduce the ability of your stomach to damage gastrointestinal cells by promoting mucosal tissue production in your digestive tract. It is also helpful in reducing intestine and stomach inflammations. Ginseng is very popular in Asian traditions because of its numerous uses. You can use ginseng to stimulate your immune system, improve your digestion, lower your cholesterol levels and prevent cancer.

Moreover, you can use spices to treat various digestive disorders. Garlic can treat duodenal and gastric ulcers, fungal infections and stomach viruses. It can help you get rid of intestinal parasites too. Turmeric or curcumin contains anti-inflammatory properties, which enables it to reduce damage caused by polyps, carcinomas, or ulcers to your gastrointestinal tract lining.

Likewise, you can use cayenne pepper to prevent duodenal and gastric ulcers as well as kill ulcer-causing bacteria. You can also use apple cider vinegar to prevent indigestion, treat heartburn and acid reflux and fight against infections. Furthermore, you can use cinnamon to fight the bacteria Escherichia coli, prevent candida growth, lower your bad cholesterol level and stabilize your blood sugar.

Chapter 6: Natural Remedies For Headaches And Migraines

In the United States, around thirty-six million people suffer from headaches and migraines. The accompanying symptoms of these ailments include intense throbbing and excruciating pain. Because of this, ninety percent of those who have headaches and migraines are not able to function normally whenever they have an attack.

If you have a headache or a migraine, you can opt for natural remedies. These remedies are less expensive and have fewer side effects compared to traditional medicines. While over-the-counter drugs are usually effective, they can also be addictive. They may even exacerbate your condition if not used properly.

One of the natural remedies you can use for headaches and migraines is lavender oil. You can either inhale or apply this oil topically. There is no need to dilute it, but you may still do so if you want. You can apply a diluted solution to your temples. However, you should never take lavender oil orally.

Peppermint oil is also ideal due to its calming and numbing properties. It actually has vaso-dilating and vaso-constricting properties that help control the flow of blood in the body. Migraines and headaches are often caused by poor blood flow. With peppermint oil, you can close and open vessels that promote blood flow.

In addition, peppermint can open up your sinuses and allow more oxygen to enter your bloodstream. You can apply this oil onto your temples and forehead to ease the pain caused by your headache or migraine. You can also use basil oil. It acts as a muscle relaxant. It provides relief from headaches caused by tight muscles and tension.

Another excellent herbal remedy for headaches and migraines is feverfew. Since the 1980's, this herb has been used to treat migraines. According to a study done in Great Britain, seventy percent of those who used feverfew daily had significantly reduced their migraines.

Feverfew contains parthenolide, a chemical that is effective against migraines. You can turn this herb into tea or eat it raw. You can also combine it with the herb white willow to increase its effectiveness against headaches and migraines. White willow has properties that are similar to aspirin.

Gingko biloba and flaxseed are also recommended for headaches and migraines. The leaves of the gingko biloba tree contain flavonoids and terpenoids. These antioxidants fight against free radicals. Flaxseed is high in omega-3 fatty acids, which can reduce inflammation that causes headaches. You can use whole or ground flaxseeds or flaxseed oil.

Buckwheat contains a flavonoid, called rutin, which counteracts cell damage. This makes it another great home remedy for headaches and migraines. You can also use ginger. It is good for digestion and it can provide relief from common symptoms of migraine such as nausea, stomachache and vomiting. Moreover, it can block prostaglandins that affect hormones, control inflammation and stimulate muscle contractions.

Chapter 7: Natural Remedies For Joint, Tendons And Ligament Ailments

Your joints, ligaments and tendons are soft tissues that allow you to move around with ease. Your muscles are the primary movers of your body. Your tendons connect your bones with your muscle bellies and help bring force across your joints to let your skeletal system move. Your ligaments connect your bones together. They are crucial for the stability of your joints.

If you encounter a problem with your soft tissues, you may resort to natural remedies. Injuries related to joints, ligaments and tendons could range from mild to severe. The level of pain, discoloration, or swelling you experience will mostly depend on the severity of your injury. Take note that mild injuries are treatable with the help of herbal remedies. You may need medical assistance if your injuries are severe.

According to Sharol Tilgner, a naturopathic doctor and expert in herbal medicine, problems with joints, ligaments, tendons and muscles can be treated with herbs that have pain-relieving and anti-inflammatory properties. Devil's claw, for instance, is a popular herb for treating tendon, ligament and muscle problems. It is also used to treat backache, arthritis and disorders related to the gallbladder, kidneys and liver.

Phyllis Balch, a nutritional consultant and nutrition researcher, states that this herb is effective in reducing symptoms of soft tissue injuries such as inflammation and pain. Aside from devil's claw, there are other herbs that contain anti-inflammatory properties. Some of them are arnica, fennel, ashwagandha, feverfew, gingko biloba, ginger, ginseng, licorice and lavender.

For herbs that help relieve pain related to soft tissues, you can choose from comfrey, celandine, goldenrod, dong quai, gotu kola, myrrh, passionflower, and kava kava. If you are suffering from arthritis, you can use a variety of herbs and plants to treat your condition. Natural remedies can provide you with relief. Just make sure that you get a clearance from your doctor first.

Aloe Vera is helpful in treating arthritis. You can get the gel and apply it to your aching joints. Boswellia, also known as frankincense, is preferred by numerous practitioners of alternative medicine due to its anti-inflammatory properties. It blocks leukotriene, elements that affect the joints in rheumatoid arthritis and other autoimmune diseases. You can use it in the form of topical cream or tablet.

You can also use eucalyptus. Its leaves contain tannins that can reduce swelling and pain. The National Center for Complementary and Alternative Medicine recommends ginger since it contains anti-inflammatory properties and can reduce swelling of the joints. The NCCAM also recommends green tea due to its ability to reduce inflammation and treat osteoarthritis.

Chapter 8: Natural Remedies For Depression

It is normal to feel sad once in a while. Going through a divorce or breakup, moving to another city, or losing a job can make you depressed. However, if your depression is starting to take over your life, you should take action immediately. While it is reasonable to seek professional help, you may also want to try natural remedies. The treatments mentioned in this chapter are effective in treating mild to moderate depression.

You can try St. John's Wort. This herb has long been used to treat nervousness, anxiousness and insomnia. A study published in the Cochrane Systematic Review stated that this herb can be just as effective as prescription antidepressants but with fewer side effects. It is also effective in treating sleep disorders, promoting relaxation and increasing energy levels.

You can also use CamuCamu. Dr. Garry Null, a renowned nutritionist and researcher, stated that it is one of the most potent plants that contain natural antidepressant properties. It also has adaptogenic properties that can alleviate stress and depression. CamuCamu berries are high in vitamin C and other nutrients that benefit the immune system, reduce inflammation, prevent herpes and fight against bacteria and viruses.

Another plant that contains adaptogenic properties is Ashwagandha. In fact, its effectiveness in relieving symptoms of stress and depression has been published in the Phytomedicine Journal. Ashwagandha also helps prevent the onset of degenerative diseases such as Alzheimer's and Parkinson's. In addition, it helps prevent cancer cells from developing and spreading.

Peruvian ginseng or Maca is ideal for treating depression too. A 2008 study showed that this herb is a natural antidepressant that can significantly reduce the symptoms of anxiety and depression in women undergoing menopause. Moreover, it can increase libido, boost energy levels and stamina and improve the immune, adrenal and endocrine systems of the body.

You can also use RhodiolaRosea. The roots of this plant can help improve both your physical and mental endurance, alleviate your depression, reduce your anxiety and boost your mood. Scientists consider it as an adaptogen because it can balance out hormones in the immune and endocrine systems as well as regulate how the body responds to stress.

Aside from herbs, you should also consume foods that are rich in omega-3 fatty acids and folic acid. Omega-3 fatty acids are necessary for normal brain function. According to studies, people with a low dietary intake of omega-3 are more prone to depression. You can get omega-3 fatty acids from cold water fish sources, such as sardines, anchovies and salmon.

Folic acid, on the other hand, is a B vitamin that is found in fruits, green leafy vegetables and beans. According to researchers at Harvard University, people who lack this B vitamin are not only more prone to depression but also tend to not respond well to antidepressants.

Furthermore, people with depression are encouraged to exercise more often. Exercise has plenty of benefits, including improving your physique, reducing stress and maintaining your mental fitness. Researchers have also found that exercise can improve your concentration, alertness and cognitive function. What's more, exercising releases endorphins, which naturally improves your mood.

Chapter 9: Natural Remedies For Sleep Insomnia

In the United States, sixty percent of Americans have sleep problems every night. The National Sleep Foundation states that thirty to forty percent of adults report that they experience occasional insomnia while ten to fifteen percent say that they have difficulty sleeping all the time.

According to Dr. Qanta Ahmed, a sleep specialist, insomnia is a complex condition that is usually caused by various factors and that these factors need to be addressed by environmental and lifestyle changes. If you have insomnia, you can try the following natural treatments to help you sleep better.

Calcium and magnesium can both help you sleep better. They are actually more effective if you take them together. Also, if you take magnesium, you can prevent heart ailments that may be caused by calcium supplements. Ideally, you should take six hundred milligrams of calcium and two hundred milligrams of magnesium every night.

Aromatherapy is also ideal. You can use lavender oil to calm you and encourage sleep. If you want to relax your mind and body before going to sleep, you can take a lavender oil bath. Just add a few drops of this essential oil to your bath water. You can also spray some of the essential oil on your pillow.

L-theanine is an amino acid that is found in green tea. It can help you stay alert during the day and sleep better at night. It works by increasing the amount of your feel-good hormones. According to a study done in 2007, it can even reduce your immune responses to stress. Additionally, it can induce brain waves associated with relaxation.

Among the most common herbal remedies for insomnia is the valerian root. Numerous studies have shown that this herb can indeed improve the overall quality of sleep. According to Dr. Tracey Marks, a psychiatrist in Atlanta, valerian has sedative properties and is helpful in making people fall asleep.

You can also use wild lettuce. It helps reduce your anxiety, makes you calmer, and relieves any joint or muscle pain, anxiety, or headaches. Hops are also recommended if you want to sleep better. The extracts from these flowers are actually used as a mild sedative for insomnia and anxiety.

Chapter 10: Natural Remedies For Sinus & Yeast Infections

Approximately thirty-seven million Americans have chronic sinusitis or sinus infection. This condition is usually accompanied by headaches, fatigue, facial pain and yellow-green nasal discharge. It can result from exposure to allergens, pathogens, weather changes and air pollution. It can also be caused by stress, dental infection, food allergies, symptoms of colds and flu, and fungal infection inside the sinus cavity.

Fortunately, sinus infection can be treated with several natural remedies and a change of diet. If you have sinus infection, see to it that you eliminate dairy products such as yogurt, ice cream, milk, and cheese from your diet to help reduce mucus production and allow your sinuses to clear. Likewise, you should avoid foods that can encourage mucus production. These foods include eggs, sugar, chocolates and fried foods.

You can also turn to herbal remedies. Herbs such as horseradish, onion, garlic, and cayenne pepper are particularly helpful in treating sinus infection. They can help dissolve and get rid of excess mucus. Horseradish can clear your nasal passages faster. You can take a spoonful of lemon juice mixed with horseradish if you want your nose to start running.

If you prefer to use a neti pot, you should dissolve one teaspoon of salt in two cups of warm water. Then, stand over your sink while you pour water into your nostril. Be careful when you tilt your head. You may accidentally reroute the water down your throat. Once you are done with one nostril, you should refill your neti pot and do the same process with your other nostril.

Apple cider vinegar has a lot of uses, including thinning congested mucus. When you first notice symptoms of sinus infection, you should immediately combine one to two teaspoons of apple cider vinegar with six ounces of water and one teaspoon of honey. Drink this concoction three times per day for five days. When your mucus has thinned out, it will be easier to eliminate.

You can also use grapefruit seed extract. It contains antibiotic properties that inhibit parasites, microbes, viruses, bacteria, and fungi. You can use grapefruit seed extract in the form of a nasal spray to treat your sinus infection. Furthermore, you can use ginger extract or ginger tea to allow you to breathe easier. Ginger contains volatile oils and pungent phenols that can act as expectorants.

For yeast infection, you can use tea tree oil. Tea tree oil has antibacterial and antifungal properties that can help eliminate the bacteria that cause unpleasant vaginal odor and itchiness. You can make a vaginal douche with tea tree oil, lavender oil, thyme oil, chamomile tea and water. Use this douche twice a day until your yeast infection is treated.

Conclusion

Thank you again for purchasing this book on Natural Remedies!

I am extremely excited to pass this information along to you, and I am so happy that you now have read and can hopefully implement these strategies going forward.

I hope this book was able to help you understand the many uses and benefits of herbs and how to use them.

The next step is to get started using this information and to hopefully live a longer and happier life!

Please don't be someone who just reads this information and doesn't apply it, the strategies in this book will only benefit you if you use them!

If you know of anyone else that could benefit from the information presented here please inform them of this book.

Finally, if you enjoyed this book and feel it has added value to your life in any way, please take the time to share your thoughts and post a review on Amazon. It'd be greatly appreciated!

Thank you and good luck!

Preview Of:

The Ultimate Feng Shui For Beginners Guide!

<u>Feng Shui</u>

Learn Feng Shui Techniques For Increased Simplicity, Health, Wealth, Happiness, And Comfort In Your Home And Life!

Introduction

I want to thank you and congratulate you for purchasing the book, *"The Ultimate Feng Shui for Beginners Guide!"*

This book contains proven steps and strategies on how to implement the principles of Feng Shui to improve your health, encourage the smooth flow of wealth in your life and promote harmony in all aspects of your life. The tips and techniques shared in this book have been simplified so that you can better understand how the principles work and how you can apply them in your own life.

Some of the techniques you will learn will aid in bringing you all the good things you want in your life while the other techniques will make it easier for you to retain those good things in your life once you got hold of them. Always keep in mind that all the techniques and strategies included in this book are founded on the basic fact that you, just like the rest of us, deserve to live a life of abundance, fulfillment, success and happiness. I hope that this book will help you live the kind of life you desire for yourself and your family.

Thanks again for purchasing this book, I hope you enjoy it!

Chapter 1: Understanding What Feng Shui Is And The Practices It Incorporates

Even though Feng Shui is a practice that has been performed in the Eastern countries for more than thousands of years, it is still considered fairly new to the western countries. A lot of Westerners may view Feng Shui as enigmatic or unfamiliar but it is in reality a quite reasonable set of both ideas and actions. When you know and practice the principles of Feng Shui, you will have the ability to create harmony, balance and comfort in nearly every environment or circumstance. Imagine having balance in all aspects of your life including your relationships and physical, mental, financial and spiritual wealth. For you start learning more about Feng Shui, you need to spend some time to reflect and seriously assess every area of your house. Go ahead and examine all the rooms and areas not only within your house but the outside, as well. It is also ideal if you already know your Kua number so you will have a better understanding of your compatible elements, colors and directions.

Chi Energy

Based on the earliest Chinese belief regarding the universe, there are a number of diverse energy sources that travel within and around us. One of those energy sources is Sheng Chi which is known to bring goodness, abundance, health and joy. You are believed to have Sheng Chi when you have a positive outlook in life and good things are continuously flowing to your life. You will know when you have Sheng Chi within and around you. You will have that comforting feeling knowing that you are in a safe and happy place where things seem light and airy. When your life and your surroundings are uncluttered and filled with plants, fresh flowers and lots of bright sunshine, you will sense the Sheng Chi energy working for you.

When it seems like things in all areas of your life are not going the way you want them and you always feel miserable, upset and angry, it means that Sheng Chi is not present in your life and you have the bad energy which is referred to as Sha Chi. This happens when you associate with the wrong kinds of people, you live in the wrong place or you connect with poison arrows that come your way. Sha chi can drain all your positive energies and replace them with negative ones that can ultimately make you ill. Sha Chi energy can also result from inhabiting in a place with underground water. A poison arrow is the corner of other houses or buildings that point at your front door or in the general direction of the area where you spend most time working. Sha Chi energy is also plentiful in places where the earth is worn-out, vegetation is meager, animals are sickly and people are broke and deprived. Sha Chi is also abundant in your life when you are feeling downhearted and depressed.

Thanks for Previewing My Exciting Book Entitled:

"Feng Shui: The Ultimate Feng Shui For Beginners Guide! - Learn Feng Shui Techniques For Increased Simplicity, Health, Wealth, Happiness, And Comfort In Your Home And Life!"

To purchase this book, simply go to the Amazon Kindle store and simply search:

"FENG SHUI"

Then just scroll down until you see my book. You will know it is mine because you will see my name "Mia Conrad" underneath the title.

Alternatively, you can visit my author page on Amazon to see this book and other work I have done. Thanks so much, and please don't forget your free bonuses

DON'T LEAVE YET! - CHECK OUT YOUR FREE BONUSES BELOW!

Free Bonus Offer: Get Free Access To The www.LuxyLifeNaturals.com VIP Newsletter!

Once you enter your email address you will immediately get free access to this awesome newsletter!

But wait, right now if you join now for free you will also get free access to the "Secrets of Becoming A Meditation Expert – In 7 Days!" free eBook!

To claim both your FREE VIP NEWSLETTER MEMBERSHIP and your FREE BONUS eBook on the SECRETS OF BECOMING A MEDITATION EXPERT IN 7 DAYS!

Just Go To:

www.LuxyLifeNaturals.com

* 9 7 8 1 5 1 5 0 6 7 1 4 6 *